Table of Contents

About Me

I have a PhD in Molecular Biochemistry and Biophysics. I have been a teacher for over 20 years. I did aging experiments for 2 years. I also did research at Argonne National Laboratory for 5 years. I wrote computer simulations for the physics of muscle contraction at the nanometer level. I developed software that used physics, mathematics, and biology. It was used to interpret x-ray images of muscles on a nanometer scale. The software gave information regarding muscle structure and details about how it contracted. I increased the efficiency of software used to study muscle contraction.

John Costello, PhD

Introduction

People suffer and die from all kinds of illnesses. According to the CDC, 635,260 people died from heart disease in the United States in 2016. 598,038 people in the US died from cancer in 2016. Stroke, chronic lower respiratory infections, influenza, and pneumonia killed 348,275 people in the US in 2016. Vitamin C in large dosages can cure or treat those conditions.

High dose vitamin C reduces or eliminates the need for antibiotics, blood thinners, antivirals, pain killers, and blood pressure medications.

Vitamin C as ascorbic acid destroys viruses and bacteria, kills cancer cells, prevents heart disease, reduces blood pressure, decreases the risks of strokes, reduces pain, inhibits HIV replication, reduces the risk of blood clots, and much more.

Vitamin C can save numerous lives from deadly infections, cancer, and heart disease; although, some people with certain conditions could have an acute reaction taking high dose vitamin C. I explain in the section labeled "Possible Negative Effects of Vitamin C". Also, I would avoid taking liposomal vitamin C because it lacks the bowel tolerance check point. I will explain in the section "Do not Take Liposomal Vitamin C". Oral vitamin C as ascorbic acid without liposomes is the form that should be taken.

I present my theory about how vitamin C destroys viruses and bacteria. It explains why vitamin C works against infections.

I started my career off by doing aging studies. I received an MS in Biology. I did studies on free radicals and aging. Afterward, I went on to receive a PhD in Molecular Biochemistry and Biophysics. I developed software to study X-rays and determined the structure of muscles at the nanometer level. I decided to teach after receiving my PhD.

I have taken large dosages of ascorbic acid for years for all kinds of problems. Vitamin C tremendously helped me throughout the years. I have taken massive dosages and beat most infections within a day. With each dose, I felt better.

Others informed me about their success using vitamin C against infections. One woman informed me that she was sick for weeks on multiple antibiotics and after taking between 10,000-20,000 mg of ascorbic acid, she finally felt better. Another woman, suffering from the 2017-2018 flu, commented that her fever finally broke on a 10,000 mg dosage of ascorbic acid. A man told me that he was going to visit the doctor, but after taking 10,000 mg vitamin C, he felt better.

Background

Claus Washington Jungeblut, MD, a bacteriologist in 1935 claimed vitamin C megadoses cured polio and published the idea. He also showed that vitamin C inactivated the diphtheria toxin. In 1937, he demonstrated that ascorbic acid (vitamin C) inactivated the tetanus toxin. He stated that high dose vitamin C neutralized toxins and was effective against bacterial and viral infections.

Frederick Robert Klenner applied Doctor Jungeblut's research and claimed to cure many of polio in the 1940s. He claimed that if massive dosages of vitamin C were used, 6000 to 20,000 mg, in a 24-hour period, that none would be paralyzed. At the Annual Session of the American Medical Association conducted on June 10, 1949, in Atlantic City, New Jersey, he presented his findings. When questioned and criticized, Klenner replied, "When proper amounts are used, it will destroy all virus organisms." He stated that you would not do anything with a few hundred milligrams of vitamin C: you needed large dosages. Others did not believe him. It seemed too simple. In science, you need to have an open mind. Klenner stated "Some physicians would stand by and see their patient die rather than use ascorbic acid because in their finite minds it exists only as a vitamin."

Linus Pauling (1901-1994), a two-time Noble Prize winner, advocated taking massive dosages of vitamin C to eliminate viral infections, heart disease, and cancer. He began advocating for vitamin C later in his life. The scientific community at first thought he was a quack. They also mocked that a biochemist gave them advice about medicine.

Linus Pauling does have credibility. He is the only scientist to win two unshared Noble prizes. He was also one of the founders of quantum chemistry and molecular biology.

Later research has supported his ideas about vitamin C. Vitamin C as ascorbic acid is toxic to viruses. In addition, it stimulates the immune systems into action against the invaders.

Recently a physician began to take advantage of the knowledge. A physician, Dr. Paul Marik, saved numerous patients near death from sepsis with massive vitamin C infusions. He commented on one patient: "Her kidneys weren't working. Her lungs weren't working. She was going to die." He further stated, "I was expecting the next morning when I came to work, she would be dead, but when I walked in the next morning, I got the shock of my life." The patient was well!

Viral infections can cause massive inflammation. Inflammation can cause organs to fail and the body to die. Vitamin C is a powerful anti-inflammatory in large dosages. In this way it can prevent death. In addition, vitamin C strengthens the immune system while at the same time reducing inflammation.

High dose vitamin C might have prevented deaths from septic shock during the vicious flu season of 2017-2018. People went to hospitals and still died. Intravenous vitamin C might have saved them.

High dose vitamin C would likely be beneficial for COVID-19 patients. Many died from a cytokine storm. Their immune systems overreacted. People developed massive inflammation and died. High dose vitamin C reduces inflammation. Vitamin C also strengthens the immune system, unlike some other anti-inflammatories.

Doctors prescribe people all kinds of antibiotics that at times fail. The antibiotics are effective against bacteria but not viruses. The antibiotics can have all kinds of negative side effects. In addition, antibiotics kill gut bacteria, which help modulate the immune system. Bacteria can become resistant to antibiotics.

Bacteria have not evolved to fight off high dose vitamin C. High dose vitamin C is useful against bacterial infections. Dr. Robert Cathcart recommended taking antibiotics with high dose vitamin C for bacterial infections. Vitamin C is sufficient for me, but everyone is different.

Vitamin C and Infections

Medical research has provided evidence for the effectiveness of vitamin C against viruses. A study demonstrated that individuals who took vitamin C had lower viral antibody levels which pointed to viral suppression.[2] Antibodies are produced by certain cells. Antibodies neutralize invaders. Decreased antibody levels could indicate a weakening infection: less invaders mean less antibodies produced to counter them. This is the conclusion of the study: "The clinical study of ascorbic acid and EBV infection showed the reduction in EBV EA IgG and EBV VCA IgM antibody levels over time during IVC therapy that is consistent with observations from the literature that millimolar levels of ascorbate hinder viral infection and replication in vitro".

Another study by Gorton and Jarvis again showed the effectiveness of vitamin C against viruses.[3] They concluded that vitamin C taken in megadoses before and after the appearance of cold or flu symptoms significantly reduced the symptoms of the population that received supplementation.

In an article, scientists who reviewed studies recommended that vitamin C be used to treat infections.[25] The authors stated that vitamin C prevented or reduced the symptoms from infections from viruses, bacteria, and protozoa. They based their conclusion on 148 animal studies. They claim that vitamin C shortens the duration of colds in humans giving credence for its biological effectiveness.

Often studies have contradictory results. They didn't consider the bowel tolerance idea. Many times, a person must reach bowel tolerance, the dose just short of diarrhea to get the most relief from symptoms; although, symptoms will often diminish with each dose. Often gas is an indication someone is close to bowel tolerance. Diarrhea is the end point. The body must be saturated with vitamin C to see maximum effects. A set dose for every subject does not consider differences in health, biochemistry, and weight. To properly access the effects, dosages to obtain bowel tolerance must be reached. The authors claim something similar. They believe dosages are often too low in some studies. When 6-8 grams per day vs 3-4 grams per day were used, a noticeable difference in results was observed. The authors further state that in 3 controlled studies, vitamin C prevented pneumonia.

In another study, patients with virus induced acute respiratory distress syndrome showed rapid recovery with high dose intravenous vitamin C.[41]

Dr. Andrew Weber, a pulmonologist and critical care specialist treated COVID-19 patients. Dr. Andrew Weber said "The patients who received vitamin C did significantly better than those who did not get vitamin C."

Dr. Richard Cheng claimed successful use of high dose vitamin C in the treatment of 50 moderate to severe COVID-19 patients in China.[45]

Several scientific studies provide evidence that vitamin C inhibits viral replication in HIV-infected individuals. One study claimed that vitamin C was toxic to cells that harbored HIV.[4] Cathcart stated that "Preliminary clinical evidence is that massive doses of ascorbate (50-200 grams per 24 hours) can suppress the symptoms of the disease and can markedly reduce the tendency for secondary infections."[5] A person can tolerate massive dosages when ill that he would normally not be able to tolerate.

Tests at the Pauling Institute showed a substantial reduction in HIV components p24, reverse transcriptase, and syncytia formation with vitamin C levels not toxic to cells attained by a human ingesting concentrations equivalent to 10-50 grams of vitamin C a day.

Normally, when a person is exposed to HIV, antivirals are given for 28 days to prevent infection. If a person does not have insurance or cannot afford the antivirals another possibility is high dose ascorbic acid. High dose ascorbic acid taken daily for a few weeks on early exposure to HIV could possibly prevent infection. The virus could be destroyed before it formed reservoirs in the body. Once the virus establishes itself in the body, it becomes more difficult to eliminate. Large dosages of ascorbic acid taken early on in any viral or bacterial infection might eliminate the infection quickly. A person would feel better because vitamin C greatly reduces inflammation and oxidative stress. It is powerful antioxidant, neutralizing the free radicals that cause pain.

Vitamin C acts by inhibiting viral replication, stimulating the immune system, and reducing oxidative stress. It directly binds to viruses: oxidizing and destroying them according to Dr. Klenner, M.D.[6] It inhibits the assembly of viral DNA and RNA. Immune system cells have high concentrations of vitamin C, demonstrating their need for it to function well. Vitamin C increases interferon production which prevents cells from being infected. It stimulates the production of antibodies and cytokines. It strengthens the ability of immune cells to ingest pathogens.

Vitamin C is a powerful free radical scavenger. Free radicals harm the body. They are generated in large numbers during illness. By neutralizing the free radicals, vitamin C reduces illness symptoms.

Immune cells incorporate large amounts of vitamin C and need much more when a person is sick. They need vitamin C in high quantities to work optimally. This puts a person in a state of deficiency when sick causing symptoms if the immune cells run low on vitamin C. The immune cells need to be saturated to receive maximum benefit. The body needs to be saturated to substantially ease symptoms. Saturation means taking enough to almost reach diarrhea. Often gastrointestinal distress occurs prior to saturation including excessive gas. Even without saturation, I often feel better with each dose I take. When ill, I often just keep taking it in dosages with water throughout the day until I develop diarrhea or are close to it. I can often sense it.

Doctor Robert Cathcart recommended taking vitamin C dosages throughout the day with water until bowel tolerance was reached when a person was ill. Bowel tolerance is the amount of ascorbic acid that a person can tolerate just short of diarrhea. He stated that the most relief of symptoms was obtained upon reaching bowel tolerance. Below is his vitamin C (ascorbic acid) dosage chart. He states "The patient tries to TITRATE between that amount which begins to make him feel better and that amount which almost but not quite causes diarrhea. " Cathcart stated that a person's tolerance for vitamin C went way up when sick. He claimed to help many sick people with large dosages of ascorbic acid.[7]

Note: 1 gram=1000 mg

USUAL BOWEL TOLERANCE DOSES:
Cathcart's Chart[7]

CONDITION	Grams Ascorbic Acid in 24 Hours	Number of Doses in 24 Hours
normal	4-15	4-6
mild cold	30-60	6-10
severe cold	60-100+	8-15

Influenza	100-150	8-20
ECHO, coxsackievirus	100-150	8-20
mononucleosis	150-200+	12-25
viral pneumonia	100-200+	12-25
hay fever, asthma,	15-50	4-8
environmental and food allergy	0.5-50	4-8
burn, injury, surgery	25-150+	6-20
anxiety, exercise and other mild stresses	15-25	4-6
cancer	15-100	4-15
ankylosing spondylitis	15-100	4-15
Reiter's syndrome	15-60	4-10
acute anterior uveitis	30-100	4-15
rheumatoid arthritis	15-100	4-15

bacterial infections	30-200+	10-25
infectious hepatitis	30-100	6-15
candidiasis	15-200+	6-25

Below is Klenner's vitamin C (ascorbic acid) therapeutic dosage chart. Klenner recommended 350 mg/kg/day divided in dosages. Klenner used much more on sicker patients.

mg. of Vitamin "C"	Body Weight	Number of Doses	Amt. per dose
35,000 mg.	220 lbs.	17-18	2,000 mg
18,000 mg	110 lbs.	18	1,000 mg.
9,000 mg.	55 lbs.	18	500 mg.
4,500 mg.	28 lbs.	9	500 mg.
2,300 mg.	14-15 lbs.	9	250 mg.
1,200 mg.	7-8 lbs.	9	130 - 135 mg.

I woke up feeling exhausted with a sore throat. I decided to try to beat it quickly with vitamin C as ascorbic acid. I started off by taking 10,000 mg right away with a bottle of water. I followed up about every hour with 10,000 mg of vitamin C. The first day, I took 100,000 mg. I felt a lot better. The next day, I could only tolerate 41,000 mg: an indication the infection was diminishing. On the third day, my bowel tolerance dropped to 15,000 mg which is close to my normal healthy level, indicating an end to the infection. I beat the infection with vitamin C as ascorbic acid. See my book chapter "Possible Negative Effects of Vitamin C": not everyone can safely titrate with vitamin C the way I did.

It was amazing how much vitamin C I could swallow without side effects. The body can tolerate a lot of vitamin C when you are ill. The key for me was to take enough until diarrhea was reached later in the day with dosages spread. The dosage every hour might be 500 mg, 1000 mg, 5000 mg, 10000 mg, etc. It was experimentally determined. If I took a dose and did not have gas or diarrhea, I increased it. I could often can tell when I began to have gastrointestinal distress that I was close to my limit.

Normally, I can only take around 12,000 mg a day to reach diarrhea. But, being ill, sometimes I consumed over 100,000 mg to reach diarrhea. Other times it was much less such as 20,000 mg or 50,000 mg. The amounts seem incredible, but the sicker you are, the more your body absorbs. The more toxic the infection, the more vitamin C that the body can tolerate. It is interesting to me that the body can tolerate so much ascorbic acid when ill. It is a hint that the body needs it. The key of the game is to reach diarrhea or come close to it; this means the therapeutic level is reached and the body is saturated.

Dr. Robert Cathcart recommended reaching bowel tolerance which is the point just before diarrhea; although, I often take vitamin C until I develop diarrhea when ill. Sometimes, by the time I develop bad gas, I feel better and stop.

Most infections I have had, I have beat fast, within a day. With some infections, it could take significantly longer to beat; although, vitamin C has always made me feel better upon taking a 10,000 mg dose: my symptoms dropped, and my energy levels increased. Also, by taking the vitamin C, even if I had an infection that lasted longer, I never got severely sick.

Whenever I begin to feel sick, I start titrating with vitamin C. I usually start with a 10,000 mg dose right away. Then, I take the dose every hour until I reach diarrhea. If after taking a dose, I don't have gas, and I am not getting better, then I up the dose until I reach diarrhea. I know that I can tolerate a lot more if I have not at least developed gas, but I always stop when I developed diarrhea. Miraculously, my symptoms often disappear within hours.

Vitamin C saved a dying man after his doctors gave up. Allan Smith, a New Zealand Dairy Farmer, caught Swine flu after a vacation in Fiji. Swine flu normally affects pigs, but the virus mutated and jumped species. He then developed pneumonia. His doctors wanted to take him off life support. His family pushed for intravenous vitamin C, and he was saved.[16] The doctors told the family not to bother because they thought vitamin C was ineffective. After pressure, they gave 25 grams of vitamin C in the evening and another 25 grams in the morning. The man dramatically improved, but the doctors refused to acknowledge that it was because of vitamin C. Another doctor saw Allen and took him off vitamin C, claiming it was a waste. Again, the man got sicker. The family had to hire a lawyer to force the doctors to administer vitamin C. They would not give much, so the family gave him oral dosages. The man was ultimately saved from viral pneumonia.

I noticed the same thing with the many physicians that I had spoken with: they all thought that vitamin C was a waste of time.

Vitamin C is effective against bacteria. High dose vitamin C would be useful against antibiotic resistant bacteria. Vitamin C was shown to be effective in killing the drug resistant tuberculosis bacterium.[1] The authors state "Here we show that vitamin C, a compound known to drive the Fenton reaction, sterilizes cultures of drug-susceptible and drug-resistant Mycobacterium tuberculosis, the causative agent of tuberculosis. "

Antibiotics have side effects, and bacteria can be resistant. Bacteria have not evolved a resistance to vitamin C.

Dr Robert Cathcart recommend patients take antibiotics with vitamin C. He stated that vitamin C increased the effectiveness of antibiotics; although, I don't take antibiotics. The vitamin C works well enough for me. Others might need them.

Vitamin C inhibits H.pylori, the bacterium that causes ulcers. In a study, scientists showed that taking 5 grams of ascorbic acid daily for 4 weeks eradicated the infection in a significant number of patients.[8] The authors state "However, in the vitamin C treated group eight of 27 patients (30%) who completed the treatment course the H. pylori infection was eradicated (P = 0.01)." Another study provides support stating that vitamin C protects against ulcers.[17]

I developed an ulcer and took large dose vitamin C whenever I had symptoms. The nausea and pain went away. The dosage I took was around 20,000 mg. The key for me, when I was sick, was to take ascorbic acid with water until I developed diarrhea or was close to it. This is when the maximum relief from my symptoms occurred. Often, I would feel better with each dose until I developed diarrhea or bad gas.

My Vitamin C Theory Regarding Infections

My theory is that vitamin C primarily destroys bacteria and cells infected with viruses by breaking down and forming hydrogen peroxide killing them. When vitamin C breaks down, hydrogen peroxide forms. Once a virus infects a cell, it takes over the cell machinery, making more viruses. The infected cells might have more difficulty neutralizing hydrogen peroxide. Bacteria might also have a problem. Normal human body cells can adapt and neutralize hydrogen peroxide. Bacteria and cells infected with viruses might have difficulty neutralizing hydrogen peroxide, leading to their demise: hence, the end of the infection.

Vitamin C and Pain

In addition to illness, vitamin C reduces pain sensations by neutralizing the free radicals that cause them. Cancer patients receiving high amounts of intravenous vitamin C no longer asked for morphine: Ewan Cameron M.D. had given his cancer patients 10,000 mg of ascorbic acid daily. A study showed that cancer patients taking high dose ascorbic acid reduced their dependence on opiates.[32]

Robert F. Cathcart M.D. claimed to eliminate his eye pain after surgery with large dosages of ascorbic acid.

I never take pain killers: vitamin C reduces the pain enough. When I injured my back, I took large dosages which took the edge off my back pain. I have keratoconus. My corneas are misshapen. I need to wear special contact lenses. At times, the lenses irritate the surface of my eyes. When I take 10,000 mg, my eye pain goes away.

People on pain killers, with numerous side effects, would possibly benefit from high dose vitamin C. Pain killers can lead to addiction; vitamin C does not.

Numerous studies have showed that vitamin C reduces pain. A review claimed that vitamin C possessed analgesic properties reducing pain in some clinical conditions.[29] Another study showed that vitamin C relieved the pain in a woman who had chronic fatigue, rheumatoid arthritis, and CNS vasculitis.[30] A study showed that between 7500 and 50,000 milligrams of vitamin C reduced inflammation in people with rheumatoid arthritis.[31] Neuroglia, severe nerve pain, was dramatically reduced with intravenous vitamin C at "2.5–15 g daily or every other day for 5–14 days".[34,35,36,37] Vitamin C (10-100 gram dosages, twice a week) administered to cancer patients reduced pain by 30-44 % in 1-4 weeks.[38,39]

Vitamin C and Blood Pressure

Vitamin C lowers blood pressure. Vitamin C megadoses significantly lowered systolic and diastolic blood pressure .[9] The study concluded, "Our study suggests an acute BP-reducing effect of high-dose IVC, particularly with dosages above 30 g, and in patients with prehypertension and normal BMI." Note the words "acute lowering". I agree: it quickly lowers my blood pressure.

One way vitamin C acts to drop blood pressure is by acting as a diuretic. It also reduces oxidative stress by acting as an antioxidant. An antioxidant neutralizes free radicals that cause damage to the body. Vitamin C also causes vasodilation, reducing blood pressure.

I have high blood pressure. My diastolic blood pressure is high, but according to a study, if the systolic blood pressure is below 140 mm Hg, there is not a significant chance of early death regardless of diastolic blood pressure.[12] My systolic normally varies between 130 and 160 mm Hg.

I don't take medications. The medications have all kinds of terrible side effects. I control my blood pressure with large dosages of vitamin C. When it is on the high end of its range, I take 10,000 mg of vitamin C right away, which drops my systolic blood pressure by 10 points within 30 minutes. I normally take it in dosages throughout the day to keep it lower.

A review provides more support for the use of vitamin C to treat high blood pressure.[18] It concludes "Vitamin C supplementation in hypertensive patients appears to possess modest effects on reducing systolic blood and diastolic blood pressure."

Vitamin C and Cancer

Vitamin C is beneficial to cancer patients. Pauling with his colleague, Dr. Ewan Cameron, demonstrated that intravenous vitamin C injections allowed patients to live much longer than the doctors predicted.[43] The terminal cancer patients taking ascorbic acid lived 4.2 times longer than the ones who did not. Vitamin C has anti-cancer effects.[10] According to another study, vitamin C administered orally and intravenously dramatically increased the survival times of the patients; although, the authors were cautious about the link to vitamin C.[42]

A study showed that if vitamin C is given in high enough dosages, intravenously, it destroyed cancer cells.[11] The researches claim that in some other studies, the amount of vitamin C given was not high enough, giving contradictory results. They said to reach therapeutic levels for cancer patients, it needs to be given intravenously in massive amounts. Another study stated that vitamin C increased cancer patient survival rates.[32]

When vitamin C breaks down, hydrogen peroxide is formed, which normal cells neutralize, but cancer cells have a hard time with it. The hydrogen peroxide kills the cancer cells but not the normal ones.

Studies support the use of vitamin C with cancer patients. A study provided more evidence for the anti-tumor effect of ascorbic acid.[20] Another study claims that vitamin C causes "faulty" stem cells that might turn cancerous to die.[24] Another study claimed that vitamin C prevented leukemic stem cells from spreading.[26] There is strong evidence, according to a literature review, that vitamin C significantly reduces the risk of developing all kinds of cancers including cancers of the oral cavity, stomach, pancreas, rectum, cervix, esophagus, oral cavity, stomach, pancreas, cervix, rectum, breast, and others.[28] Doctors conclude in another study, "In the supportive care setting, IV C given 1–3 times per week for 1–4 months in combination with oral vitamin C—for example, during post-adjuvant treatment—could improve or prevent deficiency, promote wound healing, lessen inflammation, improve qol or performance status, and potentially lessen the side effects of systemic treatment."[19]

Vitamin C and Heart Disease

Vitamin C prevents heart disease. Linus Pauling claimed that vitamin C prevented heart disease. He stated that it reduced atherosclerosis. It is a powerful antioxidant that neutralizes free radicals that damage the circulatory system. A study in the British Medical Journal (Vol 314, Iss 708, 1997) found that men who were vitamin C deficient had 3.5 times more risk of a heart attack. Another study conducted by Cambridge University in England and published in The Lancet found that people with the lowest serum levels of vitamin C were twice as likely to die compared to people with the highest levels of vitamin C in the study.

Vitamin C is a blood thinner, reducing the risk of a heart attack.

Animals that make their own vitamin C rarely have heart attacks. A mammal that makes its own vitamin C produces 1000 mg for each 25 pounds of body weight and much more when ill. Unfortunately, the L-gulono-γ-lactone oxidase gene mutated, and humans can't make vitamin C in their bodies. The gene codes for the enzyme L-gulono-γ-lactone oxidase which is necessary to make vitamin C.

Vitamin C strengthens blood vessels, reducing the risk of strokes in cases of a blood vessel bursting. It also reduces the risk of a stroke from a blood clot by making the platelets less sticky.

Dr. Hotze believes that heart disease is caused by not enough vitamin C in the diet. He claims that without enough vitamin C, plaque accumulates in damaged and inflamed blood vessels. He stated that vitamin C prevents inflammation and damage to blood vessels, so plaque does not accumulate.[14]

High levels of LDL cholesterol and triglycerides increase the risk of heart disease. 500 mg of vitamin C taken daily for 4 week significantly reduced triglyceride and LDL cholesterol levels in participants in a study.[15]

A study claimed that vitamin C slowed the progression of atherosclerosis in animal studies .[27]

Populations that eat diets rich in fruits and vegetables live longer. It could be due to vitamin C. A study stated "An increase in plasma vitamin C concentration equivalent to a daily 50 g increase in intake of fruit or vegetables was associated with a 20% decrease in risk of death from all causes, independent of age, systolic blood pressure, blood cholesterol concentration, smoking, diabetes, and use of supplements."[21] The results are incredible, if they are to be believed. A 20% decrease from death by just increasing fruits and vegetables by 50 grams a day is profound.

According to Nicola Reavley, vitamin C lowers the risk for heart palpitations.[22] Vitamin C reduced the strength of heart palpitations that I have had.

Other Benefits of Vitamin C

Since vitamin C is a powerful antioxidant, it prevents damage to the body. Free radicals are molecules missing electrons damaging the body. Vitamin C donates electrons stabilizing the free radicals, preventing damage.

There are other possible benefits of vitamin C. Vitamin C might increase energy levels in people with chronic fatigue syndrome by donating electrons.

If I have a headache, I take large dosages, which relieve the headache.

Vitamin C also reduced my dizzy spells from stress.

There are reports that vitamin C protects against neurodegenerative disorders, like Alzheimer's disease.[28]

A study reported that vitamin C supplementation to schizophrenics showed improvement in their mental condition.[28]

Vitamin C prevents damage from metal poisoning such as arsenic and lead.[28] Taking large vitamin C dosages for metal poisoning might be beneficial.

Vitamin C has been linked to lower risk of developing diabetes mellitus.[28]

Vitamin C taken at 300 mg/kg body weight/day for 4 weeks remarkably decreased the withdrawal symptoms of heroin addicts.[40]

Vitamin C reduces the side effects of chemotherapy, radiation, and surgery. Patients have less nausea, less hair loss, less pain, less swelling, and faster wound healing.

Vitamin C promotes tissue healing.[28] A friend of mine was in a motorcycle accident and took daily large dosages and felt better. People who have tissue or organ damage from an accident would benefit from taking large dose vitamin C. It could mean the difference between life and death.

Doctors stated that vitamin C would be beneficial to the sickest patients. The study concluded, "Evidence suggests that short-term high-dose vitamin C in selected patients may improve hemodynamic parameters, decrease fluid resuscitation requirements, reduce the incidence of perioperative atrial fibrillation, improve pain and potentially reduce sepsis-associated mortality."[23]

Dynamic Flow Model of Vitamin C

This model suggests that people should consume more vitamin C than recommended in dosages throughout the day to keep electrons flowing. Vitamin C donates electrons neutralizing free radicals that damage the body. The model claims that the human condition would be restored prior to its deterioration because of the mutation which caused a loss of natural production of ascorbic acid.

The dynamic flow model is antagonistic to the dose of vitamin C suggested by the RDA. The RDA recommends very low amounts: the amount depending on the group. For instance, men age 19 and over require 90 mg a day according to the RDA. The dynamic flow model suggests that people take regular vitamin C dosages throughout the day at higher amounts to bring them into a better state of health. I regularly take dosages throughout the day. I normally consume around 12,000 mg daily. I take more on days I feel worse. When I am under greater stress, I notice that I can take much more.

Do Not Take Liposomal Vitamin C

Oral vitamin C as ascorbic acid without liposomes is the form that should be taken.

When a person takes too much vitamin C as ascorbic acid without liposomes, the intestinal cells stop absorbing it, and the person develops diarrhea. This is the indication that the person should stop taking vitamin C.

Liposomal vitamin C is vitamin C surrounded by a lipid bilayer. It bypasses the intestinal check point: diarrhea. Therefore, it would be difficult to tell if you are taking too much. It is possible that someone could develop diarrhea from the lipids, but it would not indicate maximum vitamin C absorption because it would not be from the vitamin C but from the lipids around the vitamin C. For this reason, taking liposomal vitamin C is not safe.

Vitamin C should be taken as ascorbic acid without liposomes; otherwise, a person would not know if they are taking too much. Not everyone is the same; some could still have a negative reaction taking vitamin C as ascorbic acid even without liposomes. See the next chapter.

Possible Negative Effects of Vitamin C

Some people can't take high dose vitamin C: they would have a bad reaction. I have read reports where a few people had problems with vitamin C which caused crystal formation and significant health issues, possibly because of a genetic abnormality and or preexisting kidney problems.

I only found 3 reports of deaths associated with high dose vitamin C in decades of its use by numerous people: The people who died had certain conditions. One had a recent kidney transplant. Another had glucose-6-phosphate-dehydrogenase deficiency. A third person, with advanced cancer, died from massive tumor necrosis and hemorrhaging after receiving intravenous vitamin C. Slow drip IV infusion is recommended. There could be more deaths related to vitamin C that I am unaware of.

I read a report about a woman who received a kidney transplant that died after taking high dose vitamin C.

I found 3 reports about people who had a mutated glucose-6-phosphate-dehydrogenase gene who took large dosages of vitamin C and developed serious health issues. In one case, a 68-year old man died after receiving 80 g intravenous vitamin C for burns: he was glucose-6-phosphate-dehydrogenase deficient and developed acute haemolysis (red blood cell destruction). In another report, two boys in India developed acute haemolysis after binging on fizzy drinks, each containing between 4-6 grams of ascorbic acid. In a third case, a man with a history of HIV and malaria developed acute haemolysis after an 80-gram dosage of intravenous vitamin C. He was also glucose-6-phosphate-dehydrogenase deficient.

Acute haemolysis is red blood cell destruction causing symptoms such as shortness of breath, dark urine, rapid heartbeat, paleness, fever fatigue, dizziness, and jaundice.

About 400 million out of the about 7.7 billion population are estimated to have varying degrees of glucose-6-phosphate-dehydrogase deficiency. They might have a problem with high dose vitamin C.

Kidney disease and glucose-6-phosphate dehydrogenase deficiency can be tested for in individuals, but there still could be other factors or conditions that could cause serious problems for some people taking high dose vitamin C. For instance, I mentioned earlier, the case of the person with advanced cancer that died after receiving high dose vitamin C: the rapid death of tumor cells caused the death of the individual. A slower infusion of vitamin C would decrease the rate of cancer cell death and increase the survivability of the individual.

Vitamin C is also contraindicated with people blood disorders such as sickle cell disease, hemochromatosis, and thalassemia.[44]

IV vitamin C is contraindicated in situations where increased fluids, sodium, or chelating could cause problems according to Riordan Clinic.

Vitamin C might raise blood sugar.

There might be other contraindications not mentioned in this book.

Many people would not have problems. A study reported no kidney stones or change in kidney function with long-term intravenous vitamin C on 157 patients studied.[33] Dr. Robert Cathcart claimed that thousands of patients treated with vitamin C megadose therapy did not have problems except for a few who experienced minor negative effects. I have taken several blood tests over a period of years; I saw no significant difference in kidney function. A 155-pound goat naturally produces over 13,000 mg daily of vitamin C daily and much more under stress and does not have problems. According to Steve Hickey, PhD and Hilary Roberts, PhD, vitamin C does not cause kidney stones. Doctor Robert Cathcart claimed that vitamin C prevents kidney stones.

Serious side effects are less likely with oral vitamin C as ascorbic acid without liposomes than with intravenous vitamin C or liposomal vitamin C; although not impossible. The American Association of Poison Control Centers has reported zero deaths from oral vitamin C toxicity as far back as I found records. It does not mean that deaths from oral vitamin C as ascorbic acid without liposomes cannot happen. There is always a risk. People are not the same biochemically.

Concluding Remarks

I presented the case for vitamin C and treating all kinds of illnesses. I have only touched the surface. Vitamin C has potential to treat other conditions. It has worked for me and others. It can be dangerous for some people; although, I think many people would benefit from the miracle of vitamin C as ascorbic acid. It can save lives. It has helped me. If I ever feel sick in any way, I will continue to take large dose vitamin C.

References

1) Vilcheze C, Hartman T, Weinrick B, Jacobs WR Jr. Mycobacterium tuberculosis is extraordinarily sensitive to killing by a vitamin C-induced Fenton reaction. Nat Commun. 2013;4:1881. doi: 10.1038/ncomms2898.

2) Nina A. Mikirova and Ronald Hunninghake. Effect of high dose vitamin C on Epstein-Barr viral infection. Med Sci Monit. 2014; 20: 725–732.Published online 2014 May 3. doi: 10.12659/MSM.890423

3) Gorton HC, Jarvis K. The effectiveness of vitamin C in preventing and relieving the symptoms of virus-induced respiratory infections. J Manipulative Physiol Ther. 1999 Oct;22(8):530-3.

4) Rivas CI, Vera JC, Guaiquil VH, Velásquez FV, Borquez-Ojeda OA, Cárcamo JG, Concha II, Golde DW.Increased Uptake and Accumulation of Vitamin C in Human Immunodeficiency Virus 1-infected Hematopoietic Cell Lines. J Biol Chem. 1997 Feb 28;272(9):5814-20.

5) Cathcart RF 3rd. Vitamin C in the treatment of acquired immune deficiency syndrome (AIDS). Med Hypotheses. 1984 Aug;14(4):423-33.

6) KLENNER FR. Massive doses of vitamin C and the virus diseases. South Med Surg. 1951 Apr;113(4):101-7.

7) Cathcart RF. Vitamin C, titrating to bowel tolerance, anascorbemia, and acute induced scurvy. Med Hypotheses. 1981 Nov;7(11):1359-76.

8) Jarosz M, Dzieniszewski J, Dabrowska-Ufniarz E, Wartanowicz M, Ziemlanski S, Reed PI. Effects of high dose vitamin C treatment on Helicobacter pylori infection and total vitamin C concentration in gastric juice. Eur J Cancer Prev. 1998 Dec;7(6):449-54.

9) Ried K, Travica N, Sali A. The acute effect of high-dose intravenous vitamin C and other nutrients on blood pressure: a cohort study. Blood Press Monit. 2016 Jun;21(3):160-7. doi: 10.1097/MBP.0000000000000178.

10) Jiska van der Reest and Eyal Gottlieb, Anti-cancer effects of vitamin C revisited. Cell Res. 2016 Mar; 26(3): 269–270.Published online 2016 Jan 15. doi: 10.1038/cr.2016.7

11) Claire M. Doskey,Visarut Buranasudja, Brett A. Wagner,bJustin G. Wilkes,Juan Du, Joseph J. Cullen and Garry R. Buettner Tumor cells have decreased ability to metabolize H_2O_2: Implications for pharmacological ascorbate in cancer therapy. Redox Biol. 2016 Dec; 10: 274–284.Published online 2016 Oct 28. doi: 10.1016/j.redox.2016.10.010

12) European Society of Hypertension.Only systolic blood pressure drives cardiovascular risk – New paper sets the starting point for a paradigm shift. 2008.

13) Patrick J. Skerrett, MA and Walter C. Willett, MD, DrPH. Essentials of Healthy Eating: A Guide. J Midwifery Women's Health. 2010 Nov-Dec; 55(6): 492–501. doi: 10.1016/j.jmwh.2010.06.019

14) Dr. Hotze. Vitamin C for Heart Disease Prevention. Hotze Health & Wellness Center. 2019

15) McRae MP. Vitamin C supplementation lowers serum low-density lipoprotein cholesterol and triglycerides: a meta-analysis of 13 randomized controlled trials. J Chiropr Med. 2008 Jun;7(2):48-58. doi: 10.1016/j.jcme.2008.01.002.

16) Jeffrey Dach MD. Vitamin C Saves Dying Man of Viral Pneumonia: July 21, 2013

17) University Of California - San Francisco. Vitamin C May Protect Against Ulcer-causing Bacteria, Study Finds. August 1, 2003

18) Marc P. McRaea. Is vitamin C an effective antihypertensive supplement? A review and analysis of the literature. J Chiropr Med. 2006 Summer; 5(2): 60–64.Published online 2006. doi: 10.1016/S0899-3467(07)60134-7

19) Klimant E, Wright H, Rubin D, Seely D, Markman M. Intravenous vitamin C in the supportive care of cancer patients: a review and rational approach. Curr Oncol. 2018 Apr;25(2):139-148. doi: 10.3747/co.25.3790. Epub 2018 Apr 30.

20) Margreet C. M. Vissers and Andrew B. Das. Potential Mechanisms of Action for Vitamin C in Cancer: Reviewing the Evidence. Front Physiol. 2018; 9: 809.Published online 2018 Jul 3. doi: 10.3389/fphys.2018.00809

21) Jacqui Wise. Small rise in vitamin C intake could greatly reduce heart disease. BMJ. 2001 Mar 10; 322(7286): 576.

22) R. Y. LANGHAM, PH.D.. Vitamins for Palpitations.livestrong.com. 2019

23) Nabzdyk CS, Bittner EA. Vitamin C in the critically ill - indications and controversies. World J Crit Care Med. 2018 Oct 16;7(5):52-61. doi: 10.5492/wjccm.v7.i5.52. eCollection 2018 Oct 16.

24) NYU Langone Health / NYU School of Medicine. Vitamin C may encourage blood cancer stem cells to die. August 17, 2017.

25) Harri Hemila. Vitamin C and Infections. Nutrients. 2017 Apr; 9(4): 339.Published online 2017 Mar 29. doi: 10.3390/nu9040339

26) Cimmino L, Dolgalev I, Wang Y , Yoshimi A , Martin GH , Wang J , Ng V , Xia B , Witkowski MT , Mitchell-Flack M , Grillo I , Bakogianni S , Ndiaye-Lobry D , Martín MT , Guillamot M , Banh RS , Xu M , Figueroa ME , Dickins RA , Abdel-Wahab O , Park CY , Tsirigos A , Neel BG , Aifantis I . Restoration of TET2 Function Blocks Aberrant Self-Renewal and Leukemia Progression. Cell.com. August 17, 2017

27) Lynch SM, Gaziano JM, Frei B. Ascorbic acid and atherosclerotic cardiovascular disease. Subcell Biochem. 1996;25:331-67.

28) Shailja Chambial, Shailendra Dwivedi, Kamla Kant Shukla,Placheril J. John, and Praveen Sharma. Vitamin C in Disease Prevention and Cure: An Overview. Indian J Clin Biochem. 2013 Oct; 28(4): 314–328.Published online 2013 Sep 1.

29) Anitra C. Carr and Cate McCall: The role of vitamin C in the treatment of pain: new insights. J Transl Med. 2017; 15: 77. Published online 2017 Apr 14. doi: 10.1186/s12967-017-1179-7

30) Carr AC, Vissers MCM, Cook J. Parenteral vitamin C relieves chronic fatigue and pain in a patient presenting with rheumatoid arthritis and mononeuritis multiplex secondary to CNS vasculitis. Case Rep Clin Path. 2015;2:57–61.
31) N. Mikirova, A. Rogers, J. Casciari, P. Taylor. Effect of high dose intravenous ascorbic acid on the level of inflammation in patients with rheumatoid arthritis. Riordan Clinic, Wichita, USA. 2012.

32) Cameron E, Pauling L. Supplemental ascorbate in the supportive treatment of cancer: prolongation of survival times in terminal human cancer. Proc Natl Acad Sci USA. 1976;73:3685–9.

33) Melissa Prier, Anitra C. Carr, and Nicola Baillie.No Reported Renal Stones with Intravenous Vitamin C Administration: A Prospective Case Series Study. Antioxidants(Basel). 2018 May; 7(5): 68.

34) Chen JY, Chu CC, So EC, Hsing CH, Hu ML. Treatment of postherpetic neuralgia with intravenous administration of vitamin C. Anesth Analg. 2006;103(6):1616–1617. doi: 10.1213/01.ane.0000246396.64010.ee.

35) Schencking M, Sandholzer H, Frese T. Intravenous administration of vitamin C in the treatment of herpetic neuralgia: two case reports. Med Sci Monit. 2010;16(5):CS58–61.

36) Schencking M, Kraft K. Cantharidin patches and intravenous administration of vitamin C in the concomitant treatment of herpes zoster: a case report. J Chinese Integrative Med. 2011;9(4):410–413. doi: 10.3736/jcim20110410.

37) Byun SH, Jeon Y. Administration of vitamin C in a patient with Herpes Zoster — a case report. Korean J Pain. 2011;24(2):108–111. doi: 10.3344/kjp.2011.24.2.108.

38) Yeom CH, Jung GC, Song KJ. Changes of terminal cancer patients' health-related quality of life after high dose vitamin C administration. J Korean Med Sci. 2007;22(1):7–11. doi: 10.3346/jkms.2007.22.1.7.

39) Takahashi H, Mizuno H, Yanagisawa A. High-dose intravenous vitamin C improves quality of life in cancer patients. Personalized Med Universe. 2012;2(1):49–53. doi: 10.1016/j.pmu.2012.05.008.

40) Evangelou A, Kalfakakou V, Georgakas P, Koutras V, Vezyraki P, Iliopoulou L, Vadalouka A. Ascorbic acid (vitamin C) effects on withdrawal syndrome of heroin abusers. Vivo. 2000;14(2):363–366.

41) Fowler Iii AA, Kim C, Lepler L, Malhotra R, Debesa O, Natarajan R, Fisher BJ, Syed A, DeWilde C, Priday A, Kasirajan V. Intravenous Vitamin C as Adjunctive Therapy for enterovirus/rhinovirus Induced Acute Respiratory Distress Syndrome. World J Crit Care Med 2017 Feb 4;6(1):85-90.doi: 10.5492/wjccm.v6.i1.85.

42) Sebastian J. Padayatty, Hugh D. Riordan, Stephen M. Hewitt, Arie Katz, L. John Hoffer, and Mark Levine. Intravenously administered vitamin C as cancer therapy: three cases. CMAJ. 2006 Mar 28; 174(7): 937–942.doi: 10.1503/cmaj.050346

43) Cameron E, Pauling L. Supplemental ascorbate in the supportive treatment of cancer: Prolongation of survival times in terminal human cancer. Proc Natl Acad Sci U S A. 1976 Oct;73(10):3685-9.

44) StatPearls [Internet]- Vitamin C (Ascorbic Acid) Muhammad Abdullah; Radia T. Jamil; Fibi N. Attia. Treasure Island (FL): StatsPearls Publishing; 2019 Jan-

45) Richard Z. Cheng. Can early and high intravenous dose of vitamin C prevent and treat coronavirus disease 2019 (COVID-19)?. Med Drug Discov 2020 Mar; 5: 100028. Published online 2020 Mar 26.doi 10.1016/j.medidd.2020.100028